POLYMYALGIA RHEUMATICA DIET

A Beginner's 3-Step Plan to Managing PMR Through Diet and Other Natural Methods, With Sample Recipes and a Meal Plan

Patrick Marshwell

mindplusfood

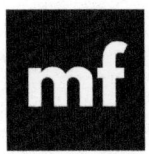

Copyright © 2022 Patrick Marshwell

All rights reserved

No part of this book may be reproduced, or stored in a retrieval system, or transmitted in any form or by any means, electronic, mechanical, photocopying, recording, or otherwise, without express written permission of the publisher.

Printed in the United States of America

CONTENTS

Title Page
Copyright
Introduction — 4
Chapter 1: All About Polymyalgia Rheumatica — 5
Chapter 2: Diagnosing and Treating Polymyalgia Rheumatica — 9
Chapter 3: Natural Methods and Home Remedies to Manage PMR — 13
Chapter 4: Managing PMR with a Healthier Diet — 17
Chapter 5: A Potential 3-Week Plan — 23
Sample Recipes — 26

Disclaimer

By reading this disclaimer, you are accepting the terms of the disclaimer in full. If you disagree with this disclaimer, please do not read the guide.

All of the content within this guide is provided for informational and educational purposes only, and should not be accepted as independent medical or other professional advice. The author is not a doctor, physician, nurse, mental health provider, or registered nutritionist/dietician. Therefore, using and reading this guide does not establish any form of a physician-patient relationship.

Always consult with a physician or another qualified health provider with any issues or questions you might have regarding any sort of medical condition. Do not ever disregard any qualified professional medical advice or delay seeking that advice because of anything you have read in this guide. The information in this guide is not intended to be any sort of medical advice and should not be used in lieu of any medical advice by a licensed and qualified medical professional.

The information in this guide has been compiled from a variety of known sources. However, the author cannot attest to or guarantee the accuracy of each source and thus should not be held liable for any errors or omissions.

You acknowledge that the publisher of this guide will not be held liable for any loss or damage of any kind incurred as a result of this guide or the reliance on any information provided within this guide. You acknowledge and agree that you assume all risk and responsibility for any action you undertake in response to the information in this guide.

Using this guide does not guarantee any particular result (e.g., weight loss or a cure). By reading this guide, you acknowledge that there are no guarantees to any specific outcome or results you can expect.

All product names, diet plans, or names used in this guide are for identification purposes only and are the property of their respective owners. The use of these names does not imply endorsement. All other trademarks cited herein are the property of their respective owners.

Where applicable, this guide is not intended to be a substitute for the original work of this diet plan and is, at most, a supplement to the original work for this diet plan and never a direct substitute. This guide is a personal expression of the facts of that diet plan.

Where applicable, persons shown in the cover images are stock photography models and the publisher has obtained the rights to use the images through license agreements with third-party stock image companies.

INTRODUCTION

Polymyalgia Rheumatica, or PMR, is a condition that causes inflammation in the muscles and joints, and in the United States alone, about 0.5 to 0.7% of the US population of adults aged 50 and older have this. That's approximately 52.5 cases in 100,000 Americans recorded annually. Usually, PMR peaks in adults ages 70 and 80.

The exact cause of PMR is unknown, but it is thought to be related to the immune system. People who have them usually experience muscle stiffness and pain. It even gets worse in the morning but improves with movement as you go about your day. For now, there isn't a specific cure for this condition but treatments to manage the symptoms are usually recommended by doctors.

One of the recommended ways to manage PMR is through diet, particularly by focusing on food that can help reduce inflammation, pain, and stiffness. The food recommendations are actually really good that even if not mainly to help with your symptoms, they are great for your overall health.

In this beginner's quick start guide, you will discover...
- The polymyalgia rheumatica or PMR condition
- Symptoms and risk factors
- Diagnosis and treatments available
- 3-week plan to manage the symptoms
- PMR-friendly recipes for your diet

CHAPTER 1: ALL ABOUT POLYMYALGIA RHEUMATICA

Polymyalgia Rheumatica (PMR) is an inflammatory disorder that causes muscle pain and stiffness. The exact cause of PMR is unknown, but it is thought to be related to the immune system. PMR typically affects people over the age of 50.

The word *polymyalgia* means "pain in many muscles," while the word *rheumatica* means "of or relating to arthritis." Inflammatory disorders are a broad category of diseases that involve inflammation. They can be caused by infection, autoimmune reactions, or other factors.

There are many different types of inflammatory disorders, each with its own symptoms and treatment options. Some other common examples include Crohn's disease, ulcerative colitis, and rheumatoid arthritis.

Arthritis is a general term for conditions that affect the joints and surrounding tissues. Arthritis is a common condition that can cause pain, stiffness, and inflammation in the joints. There are many different types of arthritis, and each has its own set of symptoms.

People with PMR typically report the muscle pain and stiffness as being worse in the morning. The pain and stiffness may improve with activity, but it typically worsens again after resting. Muscle stiffness, also called muscle rigidity, is a condition in which your muscles feel tight and unable to move. This can cause pain and discomfort. The way PMR is different is that PMR stiffness is often so severe that it can be hard to get out of bed in the morning.

The pain and stiffness of PMR can make it hard to do everyday activities, such as showering or getting dressed. In severe cases, PMR can make it difficult to walk.

Most people with PMR also experience fatigue. Fatigue is a feeling of tiredness that is not relieved by rest. Fatigue can make it hard to concentrate and make it difficult to do everyday activities.

Symptoms

The most common symptom of PMR is pain in the muscles of the shoulders, neck, and hips. The pain is often worse in the morning and improves with activity during the day.

The shoulders, neck, and hips are the most common areas affected by PMR, but the condition can also cause pain in other parts of the body, such as the arms, legs, and back. Sometimes the wrist, elbow, and knee joints may be affected.

Typically, the type of discomfort is stiffness rather than sharp pain.

In addition to muscle pain and stiffness, other symptoms of PMR may include:
- Fatigue
- Fever
- Weight loss
- Depression
- Loss of appetite

Causes of Polymyalgia Rheumatica

The exact cause of PMR is unknown, but it is thought to be related to the immune system. The immune system is the body's natural defense against infection and disease. In people with PMR, the immune system may mistakenly attack healthy tissues in the muscles and joints, causing inflammation.

One possible cause could be related to genetics. PMR tends to run in families, so there may be a genetic predisposition for the condition.

Environmental factors may also play a role in the development of PMR. For example, exposure to certain viruses or bacteria may trigger an immune response that leads to the development of PMR.

Risk factors for developing PMR include:
- Age – PMR typically affects people over the age of 50.

- Gender – Women are more likely to develop PMR than men.
- Ethnicity – White people are more likely to develop PMR than people of other racial groups.
- Family history – People with a family history of PMR or another autoimmune disorder are at increased risk for developing PMR.

CHAPTER 2: DIAGNOSING AND TREATING POLYMYALGIA RHEUMATICA

There is no single test that can diagnose PMR. Instead, the diagnosis is made based on a combination of factors, which include the following:

Medical history – Your doctor will ask about your symptoms and medical history. They may also ask about your family's medical history.

Physical examination – Your doctor will examine your muscles and joints for stiffness, pain, and inflammation.

Blood tests – Blood tests can check for markers of inflammation, such as erythrocyte sedimentation rate (ESR) and C-reactive protein (CRP).

Erythrocyte sedimentation rate (ESR), also called sed rate or Biernacki Reaction, is the rate at which red blood cells settle in a period of one hour. It is a measure of inflammation and is used as a diagnostic tool. A high ESR usually indicates the presence of inflammation.

The ESR is not a specific test for any one particular disease. Instead, it is a general indicator of inflammation. It may be elevated in a number of conditions, including infections, autoimmune diseases, and some cancers.

ESR is usually measured as part of a complete blood count (CBC). The CBC is a routine blood test that measures the number and types of cells in the blood.

To measure ESR, a small sample of blood is drawn from a vein in the arm and placed into a tube. The tube is then placed on a special stand that allows it to rotate. The rate at which the red blood cells settle is then measured.

ESR is usually expressed in mm/hr. Normal values may vary slightly depending on the age and sex of the person being tested but are generally between 0 and 20 mm/hr.

C-reactive protein (CRP) is a substance produced by the liver in response to inflammation. CRP is a biomarker of inflammation that is strongly associated with the risk of cardiovascular events, such as myocardial infarction and stroke. The liver produces CRP in response to inflammation when the body is fighting off an infection or injury.

High levels of CRP are associated with an increased risk of heart attack, stroke, and other cardiovascular events. CRP is also a strong predictor of mortality, independent of other risk factors.

The normal range for CRP is 0-3 mg/L. A high CR

Finally, imaging tests, such as X-rays or MRI, may be done to rule out other conditions that can cause similar symptoms, such as arthritis.

An MRI is a type of imaging test that uses magnetic waves to create pictures of the inside of the body. MRI can be used to diagnose a number of conditions, including muscle and joint problems, tumors, and diseases of the nervous system. The way it works is that the magnetic waves create a signal that is detected by a computer. This signal is then converted into an image.

Treatment of Polymyalgia Rheumatica

The goals of treatment are to reduce pain and inflammation, improve function, and prevent complications. PMR is usually treated with a combination of medication and lifestyle changes.

Medication

The most common medications used to treat PMR are corticosteroids, such as prednisone. These drugs are anti-inflammatory and can help to reduce pain and inflammation quickly.

Corticosteroids, in simple terms, are a class of drugs that work by mimicking the hormones produced by the adrenal glands. The adrenal glands are small glands that sit on top of the kidneys. They produce a number of hormones, including cortisol and adrenaline. These hormones are important for a number of functions, including regulating blood pressure and the immune system.

Prednisone is a type of corticosteroid that is used to treat a number of conditions, including PMR. It works by reducing inflammation. Prednisone is usually taken as a pill but can also be given as an injection.

The usual starting dose of prednisone for PMR is 10-20 mg per day. The dose is then tapered down as the symptoms improve. Most people with PMR need to take prednisone for several months before the symptoms resolve completely.

Other medications that may be used to treat PMR include:
- Nonsteroidal anti-inflammatory drugs (NSAIDs), such as ibuprofen or naproxen, can help lessen inflammation and

pain.
- Disease-modifying antirheumatic drugs (DMARDs), such as methotrexate, can be used in combination with corticosteroids to help reduce the dose of corticosteroids needed.
- Biologic agents, such as adalimumab or infliximab, are a newer type of DMARD that can be used to treat PMR.

However, many of these medications may have side effects, such as stomach pain, ulcers, or kidney problems. Be sure to talk to your doctor about the risks and benefits of these medications before starting any new medication.

CHAPTER 3: NATURAL METHODS AND HOME REMEDIES TO MANAGE PMR

In addition to medication, lifestyle changes can also help to reduce pain and inflammation. These changes may include:

- Low-impact aerobic exercises like yoga, or Chinese martial art tai chi, can help improve the range of motion and reduce pain. Yoga can help to improve flexibility and reduce pain. Yoga is a type of exercise that involves stretching, deep breathing, and meditation. It can help to improve flexibility, strength, and balance. Yoga may also help to reduce pain by promoting relaxation.

- Walking is a great light exercise that can be done almost anywhere. It's also low impact, so it's easy on your joints. And it has a host of other benefits, including reducing stress, improving heart health, and helping you lose weight. Some studies have even found that walking can improve your mood and memory. So grab your shoes and head out the door —the benefits of a brisk walk are waiting for you.

- Swimming is also low impact and easy on your joints. In addition, the water can help to support your body weight, which can make it feel easier to move. Swimming is a great workout for your whole body, including your heart and lungs. And like walking, it has a number of other benefits, including reducing stress, improving heart health, and helping you lose weight.

- Reducing joint movement or resting the joints and avoiding activities that involve a lot of movement can help to reduce pain and inflammation. For example, you can utilize a rolling laundry cart to transport laundry from your room to the washer instead of carrying it. There are also grabber tools that can help you pick up things without bending over.

Stress and Its Connection to Inflammation

Stress has been shown to be a major factor in the development of inflammation and because PMR is an inflammatory condition, it's important to find ways to reduce stress. But first, let's explore stress and its connection to inflammation.

There are two types of stress—acute stress and chronic stress:

Acute stress is the kind of stress that you feel when you're in danger or something bad happens. Your body releases adrenaline and other stress hormones to help you deal with the situation. This is known as the "fight-or-flight" response.

Chronic stress is the kind of stress that you feel when you're constantly under pressure, such as from a demanding job or a difficult home life. This kind of stress can take a toll on your health over time.

Inflammation is a natural response of the body to injury or infection. It helps the body heal by protecting against further damage and by fighting off infection. However, when inflammation persists or occurs in the absence of injury or infection, it can damage the body and lead to a number of problems, such as heart disease, arthritis, and asthma.

There are a number of factors that can contribute to inflammation, including stress. When you're stressed, your body releases chemicals into your bloodstream that can cause inflammation. This is known as the "fight-or-flight" response. While this response is helpful in times of danger, it can be harmful when it's constantly activated by chronic stress.

There are a number of ways to manage stress and reduce its impact on your health. Progressive muscle relaxation is a technique that involves tensing and relaxing different muscle groups in the body. This can help to reduce stress and improve circulation. Guided imagery is another relaxation technique that involves picturing peaceful images in your mind. This can help to distract you from pain and promote relaxation.

How to do progressive muscle relaxation:
1. Start by tensing the muscles in your toes for a count of five.
2. Work your way up to your body, tensing and relaxing each muscle group as you go.
3. Once you've reached your head and neck, spend a few minutes massaging your scalp and temples with your fingers.
4. Finally, take a few deep breaths and let your whole body relax.

How to do guided imagery:
1. Find a comfortable place to sit or lie down.
2. Close your eyes and take a few deep breaths.
3. Picture a peaceful place, such as a beach or a meadow.
4. Focus on the details of the scene, including the sounds, smells, and colors.
5. Spend a few minutes relaxing in this peaceful place.

CHAPTER 4: MANAGING PMR WITH A HEALTHIER DIET

There is no specific diet for people with PMR, but eating a healthy diet can help to reduce pain and inflammation. Some foods that may help include:

Omega-3 fatty acids

These healthy fats can help to reduce inflammation. Good sources of omega-3 fatty acids include fish, such as salmon or tuna, and flaxseed.

Omega-3 fatty acids are a type of unsaturated fat that is considered "good" fat because it is beneficial for heart health. Omega-3s can help lower blood pressure and cholesterol levels, and they also have anti-inflammatory properties.

Omega-3 fatty acids can be identified into three main types. First is the alpha-linolenic acid (ALA), which can be found in plant-based oils, such as flaxseed oil and canola oil. The second and third types are called docosahexaenoic acid (DHA) and eicosapentaenoic acid (EPA), both of which are found in fish and other seafood.

People who do not eat enough omega-3-rich foods may be at risk for heart disease, stroke, and other health problems. Omega-3 supplements are available in capsules and liquids.

List of foods with Omega-3 fatty acids:
- Fish oil
- Flaxseed oil
- Chia seeds
- Hemp seeds
- Walnuts
- Kidney beans
- Tofu
- Soymilk
- Spinach

Calcium-rich foods

Calcium is important for bone health. For PMR, calcium can help to reduce pain and inflammation. Good sources of calcium include dairy products, such as milk, cheese, and yogurt, as well as leafy green vegetables, such as broccoli and kale.

Calcium is a mineral that is found naturally in foods. Calcium is necessary for many normal functions of the body, especially bone formation and maintenance. Calcium can also bind to other minerals (such as phosphate) and aid in their removal from the body.

The Recommended Dietary Allowance (RDA) for calcium is 1,000 milligrams (mg) per day for most adults. Some people, however, may need more or less than this amount. The best way to get the proper amount of calcium is to eat a healthy diet that includes a variety of calcium-rich foods.

List of Foods with Calcium
- Dairy products: Milk, yogurt, cheese
- Leafy green vegetables: kale, spinach, collards
- Fortified foods: Orange juice, soy milk, cereals
- Beans: White beans, kidney beans, black-eyed peas
- Nuts: Almonds

- Fish with bones: Salmon, sardines

Vitamin D

Vitamin D helps the body absorb calcium. Good sources of vitamin D include sunlight, fatty fish, mushrooms, and fortified foods.

Vitamin D is a nutrient that is essential for the body to absorb and use calcium. Vitamin D is found in two forms: ergocalciferol (vitamin D2) and cholecalciferol (vitamin D3). Vitamin D2 is found in fortified foods and supplements, while vitamin D3 is found in fatty fish and exposure to sunlight.

The RDA for vitamin D is 600 international units (IU) per day for most adults, and 800 IU per day for people over the age of 70. Vitamin D supplements are available in capsules and liquids.

List of Foods with Vitamin D
- Fatty fish: Salmon, tuna, mackerel
- Mushrooms
- Fortified foods: Milk, orange juice, cereal, yogurt

Anti-inflammatory foods

These foods have anti-inflammatory properties that can help to reduce swelling and pain. For example, one property that reduces inflammation is the omega-3 fatty acids found in fish.

Examples of anti-inflammatory foods include:
- Olive oil
- Avocados
- Blueberries
- Turmeric
- Tomatoes

Foods to Avoid with PMR

There are certain foods that may make symptoms worse and should be avoided with PMR. These include:

Processed foods

These foods are high in sodium and can cause fluid retention, which can lead to swelling. These types of foods have been altered from their original state. Processing can include a wide variety of techniques, from freezing and canning to adding preservatives and other chemicals.

Processed foods are often packaged in cans, boxes, or bags. They may also come in the form of powders or bars. Many processed foods are high in fat, sugar, and salt.

These are convenient and easy to prepare. However, they often lack the nutritional value of fresh foods. processed foods may also contain harmful chemicals that can have negative health effects.

Sugar
Eating too much sugar can cause weight gain, which can exacerbate symptoms.

The reason why sugar can cause inflammation is that when sugar is metabolized, it produces advanced glycation end products (AGEs). These AGEs can damage proteins and DNA, leading to inflammation.

Sugar is a simple carbohydrate that is found in many foods. It is composed of the molecules fructose and glucose. Sugar is often added to food to sweeten it. However, sugar can also be found naturally in fruits and honey.

Too much sugar can lead to weight gain and other health problems, such as diabetes. Sugar should be consumed in moderation.

Fried foods
These foods are high in fat and can cause inflammation. Fried foods are cooked in oil at high temperatures. This type of cooking can make the fats in food more likely to cause inflammation.

Fried foods are often high in calories and unhealthy fats. They should be avoided or consumed in moderation.

Trans fats

These are found in processed foods and can cause inflammation. Trans fats are created when manufacturers add hydrogen to vegetable oils to make them solid at room temperature. These fats are often used in processed foods, such as margarine, shortening, and some types of cooking oil.

Trans fats can increase the levels of bad cholesterol in the blood and decrease the levels of good cholesterol. This can lead to inflammation.

Alcohol

Alcoholic beverages can cause dehydration and can also interact with medications used to treat PMR. Some examples of alcohol include wine, beer, and liquor. These drinks contain ethanol, which is an intoxicating ingredient in alcohol.

Alcohol can have short-term and long-term effects on your body. Short-term effects of drinking alcohol include feeling relaxed and happy, impaired judgment, slurred speech, and slowed reaction time. Long-term effects of drinking alcohol can lead to addiction, liver damage, heart disease, and cancer.

Drinking alcohol can also affect your mental health, causing problems with your mood, thinking, and behavior. If you drink alcohol, it's important to do so in moderation. Binge drinking or heavy drinking can lead to serious health problems.

7-Day Sample Meal Plan

Here is a sample meal plan made for a week that you can either follow or modify accordingly. The meals listed below are lifted from the sample recipes included in this guide. The purpose of creating a meal plan is to help you to watch what you are about to consume and make sure you're meeting your daily nutrition needs.

	Breakfast	Lunch	Dinner
Day 1	Spinach Omelet	Salmon Fry	Asparagus and Greens Salad with Tahini and Poppy Seed Dressing
Day 2	Energy Oats	Vegetable and Tofu Chili Sauté	Baked Spanish Mackerel Filets
Day 3	Blueberry Flax Smoothie	No-Fuss Tuna Casserole	Quinoa Stuffed Peppers
Day 4	Spinach and Kale Blend	Veggie Bowl	Baked Tuna and Asparagus
Day 5	Energy Oats	Ten-Minute Pasta Toss	Horseradish Aioli and Roast Beef Sandwich
Day 6	Spinach Omelet	Asparagus and Greens Salad with Tahini and Poppy Seed Dressing	Salmon Fry
Day 7	Chia Seed and Strawberry Pudding	Horseradish Aioli and Roast Beef Sandwich	No-Fuss Tuna Casserole

CHAPTER 5: A POTENTIAL 3-WEEK PLAN

Now that you have learned about the different types of foods to eat and avoid with PMR, you can start to make changes to your diet. Here is a sample 3-step plan divided into three weeks to help you get started:

Week 1: Talk to your doctor and your family
It's highly recommended that you start this journey by involving your doctor and even your family.

By consulting with your doctor first before following the diet, you can be assured that what you're doing is right, and you'll also be able to understand how exactly these changes in what you eat can greatly affect your overall health. You can also ask for recommendations about the meal plan you intend to do and follow, as well as the exercises you intend to do.

Involving your family and/or friends can also be a great way to keep you motivated and inspired to stick to your new routines. Your new routine may also push them to join you in this journey.

Remember that consulting with your doctor doesn't only happen before you start doing these things. You should regularly see your doctor so they could help you see if what you've done actually helped you or not. This way, you can also tweak the things you've done and make them more apt to your lifestyle.

Week 2: Curate your pantry

One of the best ways to start this journey is by focusing on the types of food you need to consume and avoid as you start your diet. Following the food guide listed in the previous chapter, as well as the food types recommended by your doctor or dietitian, make sure that you try to find and ask for recommendations that will surely meet your daily nutritional needs.

First, check what you have in your pantry. Try to get rid of the ingredients and food packs that fall under the category of foods you need to avoid. If you live with family, try to make them more involved in your journey. Either separate your food storage for your supplies, so you won't have to see and be tempted to eat them, or better yet, inspire your family to join you in your diet. This way, you'll be more motivated to stick to it.

Create a one-week meal plan by listing down recipes you would like to try preparing for your week one diet. You can either try out cooking new recipes for the entire week or modify old recipes to make them more applicable to what is included in your list of food recommendations.

Another tip is to do the transition gradually. There are two ways to start this—either by starting one healthy meal a day or assigning specific diet days for a week until you get used to this diet plan. That way, you can slowly adjust to the changes in your diet, as well as the new routine of being conscious in preparing your meals.

You may start by assigning three days in a week to consume only healthy foods. In the following week, make it four days a week, until you're able to transition to eating healthy food for the whole week.

The goal of this first week is to get you to be motivated in starting to live a healthier lifestyle by nourishing your body with proper nutrients instead of just eating what you want and what you're used to.

Week 3: Incorporate a PMR-friendly exercise routine
Exercising and staying active are activities that greatly benefit almost everyone. Different brain chemicals that benefit the body and mind are released when you exercise and do recreational activities that invigorate the body. Exercising also helps the mind relax and uplifts the mood.

Exercise can help reduce inflammation and improve your overall health. However, it's important to avoid high-impact activities, such as running or jumping, which can worsen symptoms. Instead, focus on low-impact exercises, such as walking, biking, and swimming. If you're not yet used to exercising, start with 10 minutes a day and gradually increase your time as you get used to it.

It's also a well-known fact that exercising greatly helps in reducing stress. Alternatively, you can also try finding other ways to relieve your stress. Most people find that doing their hobbies helps them relax their body and mind. Whether it's painting a picture, reading a book, or making handmade creations, finding means to relieve your stress will greatly benefit you.

SAMPLE RECIPES

Asparagus and Greens Salad with Tahini and Poppy Seed Dressing

Ingredients:
- 10 to 12 asparagus stalks, washed well and sliced into ribbons
- 5 radishes, washed well, and sliced thinly
- 2 to 3 rainbow carrots, peeled and sliced thinly
- 1 handful wild spinach
- 1 small handful of microgreens, washed well
- 1 small handful of sunflower greens, washed well
- Optional: few pieces of chive blossoms

For the dressing:
- 2 tbsp. tahini
- 1 tbsp. poppy seeds
- 1 tbsp. extra-virgin olive oil
- Salt and pepper, to taste

Instructions:
1. For the dressing, whisk ingredients together in a small bowl.
2. In a separate bowl, toss salad ingredients in the mixture.
3. Drizzle dressing on salad upon serving.

Quinoa Stuffed Peppers

Ingredients:
- 4 sweet bell peppers, halved vertically, with ribs and seeds removed
- 3/4 cup quinoa, well rinsed
- 15 oz. tomatoes, diced
- 4 cups basil leaves
- 10 oz. baby spinach
- 1 clove garlic, small
- 1/4 cup pistachios, unsalted
- 6 tbsp. grated parmesan cheese
- 3 tbsp. extra-virgin olive oil
- 3 tbsp. boiling water
- 1/4 tsp. kosher salt
- a pinch of black pepper, freshly ground

Instructions:
1. Combine the basil, garlic, parmesan cheese, olive oil, black pepper, and a pinch of salt in a food processor or blender.
2. Blend until the texture of the mixture appears finely chopped.
3. Stir in the boiling water.

To make the stuffed peppers:
1. Place the bell pepper halves with the side up on a lightly oiled baking sheet.
2. Roast in the oven using the high setting for about 10 minutes, or until they start to soften and have become slightly charred.
3. Remove the peppers from the oven. Set them aside.
4. In a medium pot, let the quinoa and tomatoes simmer in the vegetable broth for 10 minutes.
5. Stir in the baby spinach in small batches.
6. Scoop the quinoa-spinach mixture. Place them into the roasted peppers.

7. Drizzle the filled bell peppers with the pesto sauce.
8. Garnish with pistachios on top upon serving.

Vegetable and Tofu Chili Sauté

Ingredients:
- 1 onion, chopped
- 1 stalk, diced
- 1 carrot, diced
- 1/2 chili pepper, minced
- 2 garlic cloves, minced
- 1 green pepper, finely sliced
- 1 cup finely diced tofu
- 6 tsp. avocado oil
- 1 tbsp. brown sugar
- 1 tsp. ground cumin
- 2 cups red beans
- 1-1/2 cups of diced tomatoes
- 1 pinch salt
- 1 pinch ground pepper
- 1/3 cup grated cheddar cheese
- 4 tsp. fresh cilantro

Instructions:
1. Warm serving plates in the microwave to keep the salad warm.
2. Heat the avocado oil in a saucepan. Sauté garlic and onion for 2 minutes.
3. Toss in the vegetables. Cook for 4 minutes, stirring occasionally.
4. Pour brown sugar and toss in minced cumin and chili pepper. Cook for another minute.
5. Add in tofu and cook for 8-10 minutes.
6. Drain red and green beans and add to the saucepan. Stir well.
7. Toss in diced tomatoes and pour 1/8 cup of water, mix well. Cook for 10 minutes over low heat.
8. Add pepper and salt to taste. Pour the contents into the heated dishes.

9. Sprinkle cheddar and cilantro leaves when serving.

Veggie Bowl

Ingredients:

Cauliflower Rice and Peas:
- florets from 1 pc. cauliflower
- 1 tsp. olive oil
- 1/2 onion, chopped finely
- 1 clove garlic, minced
- 1 tsp. dried thyme
- 15-oz. can kidney beans, drained
- 1/4 cup canned coconut milk

Veggies:
- 1 large sweet potato, peeled and chopped into coins
- 2 pcs. red peppers, chopped into chunks
- 1 green plantain, chopped into coins
- 1 onion, chopped roughly into wedges
- 2 pcs. zucchinis, chopped
- 1 tbsp. olive oil
- 1/2 tsp. dried thyme
- 1/2 tsp. ground allspice
- salt
- pepper
- Optional: vegetable seasoning

Mango Habanero Vinaigrette:
- 1 mango, peeled and chopped roughly
- 1 clove of garlic, chopped roughly
- 1/4 small habanero pepper, chopped roughly
- 1 tbsp. red wine vinegar
- 1 tsp. Dijon mustard
- 1 tsp. olive oil
- Optional: fresh cilantro, chopped

Instructions:

To make the cauliflower rice and peas:
1. Pulse a third of the florets into a food processor. Process

for about 10 seconds until the florets resemble rice kernels.
2. Transfer the cauliflower rice to a large bowl.
3. Repeat until all the florets have been pulsed.
4. Heat up a teaspoon of olive oil in a sauté pan over medium heat.
5. Add the onion. Cook for about a couple of minutes.
6. Put the garlic and dried thyme. Cook for another minute.
7. Pour in the kidney beans. Stir and leave for another minute.
8. Pour in the coconut milk, followed by the cauliflower rice.
9. Cook while stirring occasionally, until the rice is slightly tender, for about 4-5 minutes. Sprinkle it with salt and pepper.
10. Once done, take off the heat and set it aside. Adjust taste if necessary.

To make the grilled veggies:
1. Toss the vegetables in a bowl or on a baking sheet.
2. Drizzle with olive oil. Add in the vegetable seasoning, allspice, thyme, salt, and pepper. Toss again to coat the vegetables.
3. If using a stove, heat up a grill pan over medium-high heat. If using a barbecue grill, heat it up to medium heat.
4. Cook the veggies in batches, until they are tender and have a nice char on the outside.
5. Sweet potatoes and plantains will need to cook for about 7 minutes on each side, red pepper for about 5-6 minutes on each side, and zucchini and onions for about 3-4 minutes on each side.

To make the mango habanero vinaigrette:
1. Place all the vinaigrette ingredients into a food processor, or blender.

2. Blend until the mixture reaches a smooth consistency.

To assemble the veggie bowls:
1. Place about a cup and a half of cauliflower rice and peas into a bowl.
2. Top it off with about 2 cups of mixed veggies.
3. Drizzle the veggies with 3 tbsp. of vinaigrette. Sprinkle with fresh cilantro if desired.
4. Serve immediately and enjoy.

Energy Oats

Ingredients:
- 1 cup rolled oats
- 1 tbsp. walnuts
- 1 tbsp. flaxseed
- 1 tbsp. almonds, sliced
- 1 cup blueberries or fruit of choice
- 1 cup almond or soy milk

Instructions:
1. Combine oats, nuts, seeds, and milk.
2. Soak for 5 minutes.
3. Microwave on medium-low for 1-2 minutes or until the oats are tender.
4. Add in fruit.
5. Serve while warm.

Horseradish Aioli and Roast Beef Sandwich

Ingredients:
- 1 tbsp. low-fat, less sodium Italian dressing
- 2 oz. roast beef, sliced
- 2 tbsp. reduced-fat mayonnaise
- 1 small cucumber, sliced
- 2 slices rye bread
- 1/2 cup fresh spinach
- 2 tsp. prepared horseradish

Instructions:
1. In a small bowl, combine horseradish and mayonnaise and stir well.
2. Put some mayonnaise mixture on each slice of bread.
3. Arrange the roast beef slices and spinach on one slice of bread and top it with the other slice of bread.
4. Serve the sandwich with slices of cucumber with dressing.

No-Fuss Tuna Casserole

Ingredients:
- 1-5 oz. can tuna, drained
- 1 can cream of chicken soup, condensed
- 3 cups macaroni, cooked
- 1-1/2 cups fried onions
- 1 cup Cheddar cheese, shredded

Instructions:
1. Preheat the oven to 350°F.
2. Prepare a 9x13-inch baking dish. Use that to mix the macaroni, tuna, and soup. Top it with cheese.
3. Bake for 25 minutes or until the casserole is bubbly.
4. Sprinkle it with fried onions. Put back in the oven and leave for 5 more minutes.
5. Serve and enjoy while hot.

Baked Spanish Mackerel Fillets

Ingredients:
- 6 pcs. Spanish mackerel filets
- 1/4 cup canola oil
- salt
- ground black pepper
- paprika
- 12 slices lemon

Instructions:
1. Arrange the oven rack so that it lies around 6 inches away from the source of heat.
2. Preheat the oven to 500°F.
3. Get a baking dish and lightly grease it.
4. Prepare each mackerel by rubbing both sides with canola oil.
5. Season the filets with salt, pepper, and paprika.
6. Top each filet with a couple of lemon slices.
7. Bake the filets for about 5 to 7 minutes, or just until the fish starts to flake.
8. Serve the fish right away.

Salmon Fry

Ingredients:
- salmon
- 1/2 tsp. smoked paprika
- 1/2 tsp. garlic powder

Instructions:
1. Coat the salmon with some garlic powder and paprika. Use other herbs if desired.
2. Place the salmon into the air fryer basket
3. Set the temperature of the Air Fryer to 400°F and cook for 10 minutes.
4. Serve and enjoy while hot.

Baked Tuna and Asparagus

Ingredients:
- 2 5-oz. tuna fillets
- 14 oz. young potatoes
- 8 asparagus spears, trimmed and halved
- 2 handfuls of cherry tomatoes
- 1 handful fresh basil leaves
- 2 tbsp. extra-virgin olive oil
- 1 tbsp. balsamic vinegar

Instructions:
1. Heat oven to 428°F.
2. Arrange potatoes in a baking dish. Drizzle with a tablespoon of extra-virgin olive oil.
3. Roast potatoes for 20 minutes, or until golden brown.
4. Place the asparagus into the baking dish together with the potatoes. Roast in the oven for another 15 minutes.
5. Arrange the cherry tomatoes and tuna among the vegetables. Drizzle with balsamic vinegar and the remaining olive oil.
6. Roast for 10 to 15 minutes, or until tuna is cooked.
7. Throw in a handful of basil leaves before transferring everything to a serving dish. Serve while hot.

Ten-Minute Pasta Toss

Ingredients:
- 16 oz. rotini pasta
- 1-1/4 tsp. garlic powder
- 4 tbsp. olive oil
- 1-1/4 tsp. dried basil
- 4 pcs. chicken breast, skinless, boneless, and cut in halves
- 1-1/4 tsp. dried oregano
- 3 cloves minced garlic
- 1 cup sun-dried tomatoes, finely chopped
- 1-1/4 tsp. salt
- 1/4 cup parmesan cheese, finely grated

Instructions:
1. Boil a large pot of salted water. Cook the rotini pasta for about 8 minutes. Drain.
2. Sauté chicken, salt, garlic, garlic powder, oregano, and basil in a preheated pot over medium-high heat for about 10 minutes.
3. Add the tomatoes and cook for a couple of minutes.
4. Remove from heat. Pour the cooked rotini pasta into the pot with sauce and toss until well combined.
5. Serve with parmesan cheese on top.

Spinach Omelet

Ingredients:
- 2 egg whites
- 1 egg
- 1/2 cup fresh spinach

Instructions:
1. Put together beaten egg and egg whites, whilst forming a "pocket-like" shape.
2. Load the pocket with spinach. Cook until the spinach is wilted. Season with salt and pepper.
3. Serve immediately.

Chia Seed and Strawberry Pudding

Ingredients:
- 1 cup strawberries, thinly sliced
- 3 tbsp. chia seeds
- 1 cup soy beverage, unsweetened and fortified

Instructions:
1. To create pudding, combine the soy beverage and chia seeds. Refrigerate the mixture for half an hour. Stir the mixture every 5 minutes to prevent the chia seeds from sticking together.
2. As an alternative, blend the soy beverage and chia seeds in a food processor and let it chill in the refrigerator.
3. Slice strawberries lengthwise.
4. Pour chilled pudding into 2 glasses. Place the strawberry slices on top.
5. Serve and enjoy your pudding.

Spinach and Kale Blend

Ingredients:
- 1 cup spinach
- 1 cup chopped kale
- 3/4 cup water
- 1/2 cup chopped cucumber
- 1 green apple
- 1 cup chopped papaya
- 1 tbsp. ground flaxseed

Instructions:
1. Using a blender, mix water, spinach, and kale. Increase speed until all solid particles are gone.
2. Add the rest of the ingredients. Resume blending until reaching the maximum speed.
3. Maintain the maximum speed for 30 seconds before serving.
4. Serve chilled.

Blueberry Flax Smoothie

Ingredients:
- 1 cup blueberries, frozen
- 1 tbsp. flaxseed, ground
- a handful of spinach leaves
- 1/4 cup full-fat Greek yogurt
- 1 cup coconut milk or any kind of milk

Instruction:

Place all ingredients in a blender or magic bullet. Mix until smooth.

Conclusion

As shown, PMR is a serious condition that can have a negative impact on your life. It's important to be aware of the symptoms and seek medical help if you think you may have the condition. There are treatments available that can help to reduce the symptoms and improve your quality of life.

There are also certain lifestyle changes that can help, such as eating a healthy diet, getting regular exercise, and avoiding processed foods.

If you think you may have PMR, talk to your doctor. They can help to diagnose the condition and recommend the best course of treatment. Take care and stay healthy. If you enjoyed this guide, please share it with others who may find it helpful and leave a review.

References and Helpful Links

4 Tips On How To Best Cope with Polymyalgia Rheumatica (PMR)... | Tristate Arthritis & Rheumatology. 25 Sept. 2021, https://www.tristatearthritis.com/polymyalgia-rheumatica-pmr/4-tips-on-how-to-best-cope-with-polymyalgia-rheumatica-pmr/. Accessed 27 June 2022.

MD, Judith Frank. "Diet and Supplements for Polymyalgia Rheumatica (PMR)." Arthritis-Health, https://www.arthritis-health.com/blog/diet-and-supplements-polymyalgia-rheumatica-pmr. Accessed 27 June 2022.

Polymyalgia Rheumatica. https://www.rheumatology.org/I-Am-A/Patient-Caregiver/Diseases-Conditions/Polymyalgia-Rheumatica. Accessed 27 June 2022.

Polymyalgia Rheumatica Diet: Foods to Eat and Avoid. 30 Apr. 2018, https://www.medicalnewstoday.com/articles/321683. Accessed 27 June 2022.

Polymyalgia Rheumatica: Practice Essentials, Pathophysiology, Etiology. Jan. 2022. eMedicine, https://emedicine.medscape.com/article/330815-overview. Accessed 27 June 2022.

UpToDate. https://www.uptodate.com/contents/clinical-manifestations-and-diagnosis-of-polymyalgia-rheumatica. Accessed 27 June 2022.

Printed in Great Britain
by Amazon